Amel BEN HAMAD
Manel CHARFI
Fatma MAGDICH

Ischemic stroke in newborns

Amel BEN HAMAD
Manel CHARFI
Fatma MAGDICH

Ischemic stroke in newborns

Risk factors and management

ScienciaScripts

Cover image: www.ingimage.com

This book is a translation from the original published under ISBN 978-620-6-72336-3.

Publisher:
Sciencia Scripts
is a trademark of
Dodo Books Indian Ocean Ltd. and OmniScriptum S.R.L publishing group

120 High Road, East Finchley, London, N2 9ED, United Kingdom
Str. Armeneasca 28/1, office 1, Chisinau MD-2012, Republic of Moldova, Europe
Printed at: see last page
ISBN: 978-620-8-34028-5

Contents

List of abbreviations

AAP : Antiplatelet agents ACC : Circulating anticoagulants
ACCP : "*American College of Chest Physicians*" Acl: anticardiolipin antibodies
AT : Antithrombin

AVCi : Ischemic stroke CID: Right internal carotid artery
DIC : Disseminated intravascular coagulation HCM: Hypertrophic cardiomyopathy
CRP: "*C-Reactive Protein*" ECG: Electrocardiogram EEG: Electroencephalogram
ETF : Transfontanellar ultrasound FVL: Factor V Leiden
IR: Rosner index

MRI: Magnetic resonance imaging of the brain

ISTH*: International Society on Thrombosis and* Haemostasis LA: Anticoagulant lupus
Lp 'a' : Lipoprotein 'a

IUFD: Intrauterine fetal death

VTE: Venous thromboembolism MTHFR: Methylenetetrahydrofolate reductase CBC: Blood cell count
OR: Odds ratio

PC : Protein C

PS : Protein S

IUGR: Intrauterine growth retardation

RPCa:Activated protein C resistance

RPM: Rupture prématurée et prolongée des membranes (premature and prolonged rupture of membranes) SAPL: Syndrome des antiphospholipides (antiphospholipid syndrome)
APTT: Activated partial thromboplastin time CT: Computed tomography
β2GPI : Beta-2-glycoproteins I

INTRODUCTION

nfant ischemic stroke is the result of an interruption in blood flow to a major cerebral artery due to embolism or thrombosis **[1]**. Infantile strokes are 10 to 12 times rarer than in adults, with an estimated incidence of 3.3 per 100,000 births **[2]**.

Perinatal stroke is the most common form of stroke, and is the leading cause of cerebral palsy and the second most common cause of neonatal convulsions after anaxo-ischemic encephalopathy **[3]**. Its clinical presentation is not very specific. Diagnosis is essentially radiological. In most cases, the diagnosis is made on the basis of a brain imaging scan ordered in response to neurological warning signs, in particular neonatal convulsions.

To this day, the pathophysiological mechanism of neonatal stroke remains debated. Indeed, multiple maternal and fetal risk factors have been identified, but their causal link with thromboembolic events remains difficult to establish **[4]**.

Several studies have demonstrated that thrombophilia marker abnormalities in children and their parents are responsible for stroke. This justifies a full etiological investigation.

Following a neonatal stroke, the child's development may be complicated by various motor and cognitive sequelae. Motor deficits may manifest themselves in children during the first few months as cerebral palsy. The aim of early rehabilitation through physiotherapy, occupational therapy or psychomotricity (separately or in combination) is to maintain joint amplitudes and avoid orthopedic deformities.

Secondly, these measures must be combined with a more global intervention with the child, enabling him to carry out his activities and, above all, to integrate socially despite his deficit syndrome.

DEFINITION

I- DEFINITION OF NEONATAL ISCHEMIC STROKE

Neonatal stroke is a heterogeneous group of diseases characterized by focal interruption of cerebral blood flow, occurring between 20ème weeks of fetal life and 28ème days post-natal. Positive diagnosis is confirmed by brain imaging or anatomopathological studies **[5]**.

Three sub-categories are then defined:

- **Fetal cerebral infarction**, diagnosed before birth by antenatal imaging or neuropathological studies in stillborn babies.
- **Neonatal cerebral infarction**, giving rise to neurological symptoms and diagnosed between birth and 28ème days of life.
- **Presumed perinatal cerebral infarction**, the diagnosis is made in children over 28 days of age in whom it is assumed that the ischemic event occurred between 20ème weeks of fetal life and the 28th postnatal day **[6]**.

EPIDEMIOLOGY

II- EPIDEMIOLOGY

The prevalence of arterial stroke in newborns at or near term is estimated at between 6 and 25 per 100,000 births **[7,8]**.

These account for approximately 80% of all strokes in term newborns. The remaining 20% are due to both cerebral venous thrombosis and cerebral haemorrhage **[9]**.

Neonatal stroke is the most frequent form of pediatric stroke. It is second only to adult stroke **[10]**.

However, its exact incidence remains ambiguous. This is explained by the absence of national registries, apart from a few countries such as Canada (the Canadian Pediatric Ischemic Stroke Registry), where incidence has been estimated at 10.2 per 100,000 live births **[7]**. Elsewhere, incidence has been estimated on the basis of rare population-based cohort and hospital studies, which explains the heterogeneity of results (**Table I**).

Table I: Main studies assessing the mean incidence

Authors	Study period	Country	Incidence 1 /x NV	Frequency per 100,000 births
Oueslati (2013) [52]	1998-2011	Tunisia	1 /4219	23
Dunbar et al. (2017) [10]	2008-2017	Canada	1/3000	33,4
Machado et al (2015) [91]	2007-2011	Portugal	1/3985	25
Gruntet al. (2015) [92]	2000-2010	Switzerland	1/5882	17

Sex ratio

A predominance of males has been reported by the majority of authors (**tableII**). Indeed, the International Pediatric Stroke Study data registry reported an average sex ratio of 1.4 **[11]**.

Table II: Sex ratio of neonatal stroke in different studies

Authors	Country	NN included	Boys	Girls	Sex ratio
Oueslati [52]	Tunisia	6	3	3	1
Shalta et al [55]	Egypt	20	14	6	2,3
deVeber et al [8]	Canada	232	128	104	1.3
López-Espejo et al [89]	Chile	33	21	12	1,75
Salih et al [93]	Saudi Arabia	63	34	29	1,17
Martinez-Biarge et al [94].	England	79	58	21	2,8

PATHOPHYSIOLOGY

III- PATHOPHYSIOLOGY

1- Physiology of neonatal cerebral circulation

The metabolic needs of the developing neonatal brain are very great, and this is expressed by the neonatal cerebral circulation, which receives 1/3 of the cardiac blood, although this value does not exceed 1/6 in adults **[12]**. What is specific to the neonatal cerebral circulation is the immaturity of the autoregulatory system. Autoregulation is the physiological mechanism that keeps cerebral blood flow relatively constant in response to changes in cerebral perfusion pressure. This regulation is dependent on the vasoconstriction and vasodilation capacities of the cerebral arteries. Thus, a decrease in cerebral blood flow can be observed following hypocapnia or arterial hypotension, exposing infants to the risk of ischemia **[13]**.

2- Pathophysiology and mechanisms of neonatal cerebral infarction

In the case of neonatal stroke, the mechanism and causes of arterial ischemia remain, in the majority of cases, at the hypothesis stage. Apart from a few obvious clinical situations (disseminated intravascular coagulation (DIC), cardiac surgery, interventional catheterization, dystocic delivery), it is difficult to determine the exact pathophysiological mechanism **[14]**. The Virchow triad describes three factors involved in thrombosis. These are: blood stasis, endothelial damage and hypercoagulability (**figure 1**) **[15]**.

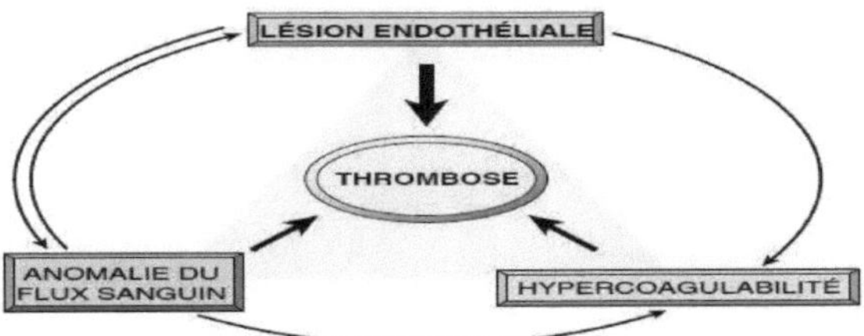

Figure 1: Virchow's triad in thrombosis [16].

Interruption of flow in a large arterial trunk may be due to in situ thrombosis, embolism or spasm of sufficient severity to cause either lasting obstruction or thrombosis-generating parietal lesions **[17]**. These often overlapping mechanisms have been identified as responsible for this pathology.

1-1- Arterial thrombosis

It is caused by damage to the arterial wall, whether or not promoted by physical or biological factors **[18]**.

1-2- Embolus

This mechanism is suggested by the specificities of feto-placental hemodynamics, favoring communications between the venous and arterial systems **[19]**. Blood flow in the brain of the newborn at term is higher than in other areas, and is supplied predominantly by the carotid arteries, which are the preferred site for stroke.

An embolus of placental origin will follow the same pathway from the fetal bloodstream to the brain: oxygenated blood is preferentially directed via the umbilical vein and then the inferior vena cava to the left ventricle, then the ascending aorta and carotid arteries through the foramen ovale (**figure 2**) **[20]**.

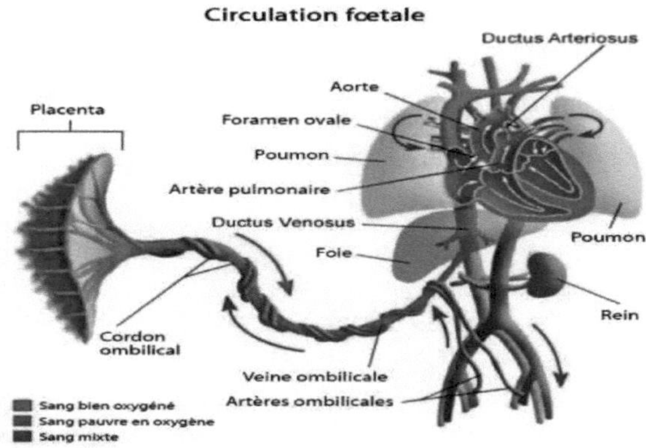

Figure 2: Representation of the feto-placental circulation [21].

1-3- Arterial dissection

These are traumatic injuries. Indeed, childbirth is an event subject to sometimes severe mechanical stress on the cervicocephalic sphere. The resulting lesions typically lead to arterial dissections. Alteration of the vascular wall leads to functional changes in the endothelium: increased cell adhesion (leukocyte and platelet adhesion), increased capillary permeability and a procoagulant state of the endothelium **[22]**.

1-4- Arterial spasm

It can occur following acute fetal distress, when major ischemia-anoxia lesions focus on one or more preferential vascular territories. The use of powerful vasoconstrictors, and abrupt changes in blood pressure or oximetry, may be accompanied by vasoconstriction and consequent vascular spasm, leading to cerebral hypoperfusion **[23]**.

1-5-Outer vascular compression

Traumatic delivery can cause stroke in the newborn by arterial compression through a large haematoma following subdural haemorrhage **[22]**.

CLINICAL PICTURE

IV- CLINICAL PICTURE

The first symptoms of stroke appear within the first week of life (within the first three days for 90% of children). Neonatal convulsions are the most frequent clinical signs **[23]**.

In the majority of cases, there is no history of poor adaptation to extra-uterine life, and most often the newborns are asymptomatic and have rejoined their mother after delivery.

Seizures are focal in 60% of cases, and one-third of these have progressed to a convulsive malaise state. These convulsions are frequently hemicorporeal clonic, contralateral to the infarcted region. The middle cerebral artery and posterior cerebral artery are often involved in strokei presenting wh hemicorporeal convulsions. In less than 10% of cases, seizures are non-motor. These are mainly apnea and/or cyanosis episodes **[24]**.

Seizures can be frustrating or atypical: chewing and sucking movements, fixed gaze, ocular revulsion, eyelid blinking, vertical nystagmus or simple hiccups.

Other non-specific symptoms may include bradycardia, hypotonia, altered consciousness or even lethargy.

Clinical examination rarely reveals lateralization of signs, with asymmetry of spontaneous movements or archaic reflexes. Hemiplegia in the neonatal period is rare and only appears later in life **[25]**.

RISK FACTORS

V- RISK FACTORS

Cerebral artery occlusion in the term newborn is not the result of a single risk factor, but is a multifactorial event arising from the interaction of several acquired or constitutional determinants of the disease at the level of each of the three main actors: the fetus, the mother and the placenta **[17,26]**.

Neonatal stroke is a pathology of multifactorial origin, with a highly complex pathophysiological mechanism. As a result, the list of risk factors continues to grow from study to study, and cannot be exhaustive.

1- Maternal and obstetrical risk factors

1-1-Maternal history and habits

History of thromboembolic disease: The presence of factor V Leiden polymorphism (FVL) and antiphospholipid antibodies imothers increases the predisposition of children to stroke **[27]**.

Arnaez et al. noted a thrombotic history frequency of 33% **[28]**. The literature also shows a high frequency of primiparity of around 25%. Indeed, the frequency of primiparity exceeded 65% in some studies, such as that by Martinez et al. (**Table III) [17]**.

Table III: Maternal characteristics and history in the various studies

	Arnaez et al [28]	Martinez et al [94]	Renaud [5]
Average age of mother	33 (20-44)	31 (27-36)	28 (22-38)
Primiparity	31%	66%	57%
Thrombotic family history	33%	15%	17%
Miscarriage	14%	24%	16%

- **A history of infertility or spontaneous miscarriage** may be associated with the presence of neonatal stroke **[34]**.

The frequency of repeated spontaneous miscarriage varies from 14% to 24% **[5,28]**.

- **Maternal autoimmune diseases** such as lupus erythematosus may result in increased plasma levels of anti-fibrinolytic agents **[30]**.
- **Maternal smoking and drug addiction** are incriminated since the vasoconstriction may affect feto-placental vascularization **[31]**.

1-2-Pregnancy conditions and pathologies

The obstetrical risk factors reported in the literature are numerous**.** to the studies in the literature (**Table I**).

Acute fetal distress is the leading gravidic risk factor in the findings of Chabrier et al., with a percentage of 33% **[33]**.

Table IV: Pregnancy conditions and pathologies in various studies

	Sorg et al [33]	Martinez et al [94]	Chabrier et al [33]
Twin pregnancies	6,7%		5%4%
Gestational diabetes	9,7%	-	7%
Pre-eclampsia	8%		9%4%
Premature and prolonged rupture of membranes	15%		21%6%
Acute fetal distress	18,8%		14%33%

This result is similar to that of Sorg et al. with a percentag[**33**]. Several case-control studies have defined emergency caesarean delivery as a risk factor for iStroke, with an OR =5.9 **[8]**.

- **Primiparity** has been identified in 30% to 75% of stroke cases in newborns **[26].**
- **Twin pregnancies** increase the risk of ischemia through the passage of microemboli between the two fetal circulations and through transfusion-transfusion syndrome **[39]**.
- **Intrauterine growth retardation (IUGR)** has been observed in several affected newborns. IUGR is accompanied by hyperviscosity, which increases the risk of hypercoagulability **[40]**.
- **Maternal infection** has often been associated with the development of stroke. The mechanism was the occurrence of DIC following an acquired prothrombotic state **[36]**.
- **Prolonged premature rupture of the membranes (RPM)** exposes the mother and fetus to the infectious risk of chorioamniotitis and fetal inflammatory syndrome **[32]**.
- **Preeclampsia and eclampsia** is a vascular-placental pathology. It

represents a considerable risk factor **[36]**.

Gestational diabetes can increase the risk of perinatal stroke through fetal polyglobulin and fetal macrosomia **[33]**. Gestational diabetes, pre-eclampsia and premature and prolonged rupture of membranes are noted with a frequency of 10%. These results are comparable to those found in a recent large German study **[41]**.

- **Maternal-fetal hemorrhage** is also a cause of perinatal stroke.

Placental damage, hypotension and hypovolemia lead to cerebral hypoperfusion and infarction **[38]**.

1-3-Circumstances of delivery

- **Traumatic delivery** is defined by the presence of one of the following situations: breech presentation, shoulder dystocia, fetopelvic disproportion or fetal macrosomia **[5,8]**. It is a source of stretching and damage to the vessels of the neck, especially the vertebral artery **[35]**.
- **Perinatal asphyxia** is classified as one of the most common risk factors

The most important risk factor for perinatal stroke is arterial spasm [Erreur ! Source du renvoi introuvable]. Erinatal asphyxia is one of the risk factors for neonatal stroke most frequently reported in the literature, with an OR ranging from 7 to 22 depending on the study **[8, 37]**. In the series by Munoz et al., the Apgar score at 5 min was less than 7, with a frequency of 10% **[38]**.

2- Neonatal risk factors

In addition to these factors , neonatal pathologies are significantly associated with the occurrence of strokei

- **Macrosomia:** the literature describes a risk ranging from 6% to 18%.

[33].

- **Congenital heart disease**: the persistence of shunts allows venous emboli to pass into the cerebral arterial circulation **[37]**.

- **Newborn infection,** mainly sepsis and meningitis, can cause neonatal stroke through inflammatory and prothrombotic mechanisms **[40]**. The case-control study by Hartemen et al. demonstrated that early onset of sepsis or meningitis is significantly associated with neonatal stroke **[42]**.
- **neonatal intensive care**, such as the use of arterial and venous catheters and extracorporeal membrane oxygenation **[18]**.
- Acquired or constitutional **coagulation disorders** are important prothrombotic risk factors **[41,43]**.

We were therefore interested in the implication of hereditary thrombophilia on the occurrence of strokei.

2-1- Definition and physiology of thrombophilia

Thrombophilia is an inherited or acquired abnormality of hemostasis that predisposes to thrombosis. Hemostasis is a set of mechanisms designed to prevent spontaneous bleeding and stop hemorrhage occurring when the vascular wall ruptures. It takes place in three stages: primary hemostasis, coagulation and fibrinolysis **[44]**.

Primary hemostasis is the set of mechanisms that lead to the formation of the platelet plug. Following a vascular lesion, platelets adhere to the vascular endothelium and aggregate to form a cluster that obstructs the breach.

Coagulation is a cascade of reactions involving coagulation factors, enzymes and fibrinogen to form the red thrombus (**figure 3)**. Thus, fibrinolysis is an enzymatic process leading to the dissolution of fibrin and subsequent lysis of the clot, thus preventing its extension **[45]**.

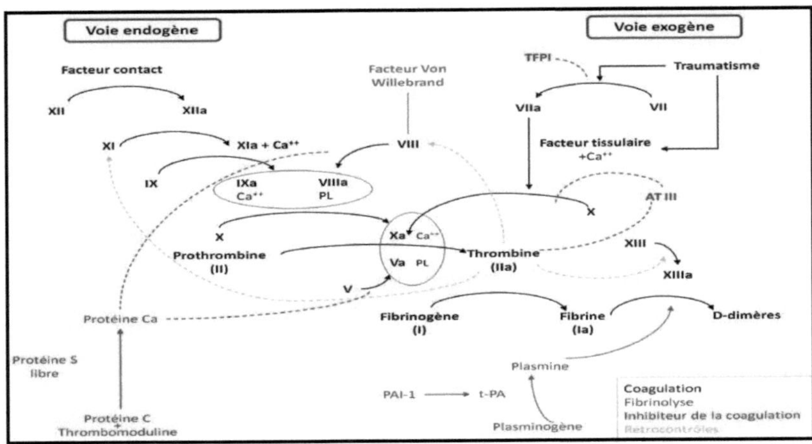

Figure 3: Coagulation diagram [45].

Several regulatory factors are involved in limiting local clot extension and diffusion. Physiological inhibitors of coagulation include antithrombin (AT), protein S (PS) and protein C (PC). Thrombophilia occurs when one of these factors is deficient. Certain genetic mutations, such as the factor II G20210 gene mutation, the FVL G1691A polymorphism and the MTHFR gene polymorphism, are the main inherited risk factors involved in stroke **[46]**.

Gestation is a particularly high-risk period for both mother and newborn, physiologically inducing a state of hypercoagulability, mainly due to the lowered coagulant activity of protein S and the increased activity of factor V, factor VIII and fibrinogen. This is a natural pre-thrombotic state. There is also a modification of platelet-vessel interaction, an increase in thrombin formation and a decrease in physiological thrombolysis **[5,47]**.

This state of hypercoagulability is also linked to altered platelet interaction with the vascular endothelium, increased thrombin formation and reduced physiological thrombolysis **[48]**.

2-2- Deficiency of physiological coagulation inhibitors

- **PS deficit**

PS is synthesized by the liver under the influence of vitamin K.

It acts as a CP cofactor in the inactivation of activated factors V and VIII **[49]**.

In a Lebanese study, Muwakkit et al. reported suspicious PS deficits in three patients who were regularized at follow-up **[50]**. Munoz et al. also failed to note PS deficiency in their study population **[38]**. According to the literature, a large series of studies revealed a higher frequency of PS deficiency, but it was still low: deVeber et al. **[7]** reported a prevalence of this deficiency of 4%. Curtis et al **[51]** reported a percentage of 12% of PS-deficient patients. In each of these studies, no significant association was established between PS deficiency and neonatal stroke.

- **PC deficit**

PC is a vitamin K-dependent anticoagulant protein. The PC-PS system neutralizes activated factors V and VIII, thereby slowing thrombin generation **[49]**.

Studies by Simchen et al. found 19% PC deficiency in their study populations **[27]**. In a Tunisian series of 6 cases, PC deficiency was identified as the main constitutional coagulation anomaly responsible for neonatal stroke. **[52]**. Moreover, several studies have revealed very low percentages of PC deficiency varying between 0.5 and 4% **[53, 54]**.

➢ AT deficiency

AT is a major physiological anticoagulant. It is a glycoprotein whose role is to neutralize thrombin and other coagulation factors (VII, IX, X). For optimal activity, AT binds to heparin sulfate, which is derived from endothelial cells **[49]**.

Deficiencies in physiological coagulation inhibitors are associated with an increased risk of thrombosis. These deficiencies were observed in 4.7% of newborns with stroke **[53]**.

Shalta et al. and Kurnik et al. reported an absence of AT deficiency **[55, 56]**. However, a low percentage of AT deficiency (0.4%) was noted in the meta-analysis by Perez et al **[57]**.Nevertheless, a large study carried out on an international population showed an association between the frequency of AT deficiency, the coexistence of more than one prothrombotic factor and an increased risk of stroke (**Table V**) **[58]**.

Table V: Coagulation inhibitor deficiency in neonatal ischemic stroke

series	PS deficit % (n/N)	PC deficit % (n/N)	AT deficit % (n /N)
Oueslati [52]	0	50% (3 /6)	-
Curtis et al [51]	12% (9/76)	9% (7/76)	1% (1/76)
Deveber et al [58]	4% (28/708)	3,3% (26/778)	3,1% (23/750)
Duran et al [78]	0	10% (3/30)	6,7% (2/30)

This difference in coagulation inhibitor deficiency frequencies can be explained by the particularity of hemostasis in the newborn. Indeed, the balance of hemostasis is fragile in the newborn, who is exposed to acquired and constitutional pathologies of hemostasis, sometimes severe. The diagnosis of deficiencies is sometimes difficult in the newborn, due to the physiologically very low levels of certain coagulation inhibitors **[59]**.

2-3- Factor V Leiden G1691A polymorphism

FVL is the genetic confirmation of resistance to activated protein C (RPCa). Activated PC is responsible for the inactivation of activated factor V during the coagulation cascade. The presence of the FVL G1691A polymorphism would prevent this inactivation and thus lead to thrombus formation **[60]**. FVL results from a single nucleotide mutation, manifested by a replacement of the adenine base by guanine at position G1691A of factor V **[61]**. This is the most frequent anomaly in hereditary thrombophilias (4-10% of the general population) **[62]**. The Turkish series by Duran et al. revealed a frequency of 23.3% of children with iCVA having this polymorphism. The meta-analysis by Kenet et al. including 22 studies and 1014 patients, revealed a strong link between LVF polymorphism and stroke: OR=3.70 95% CI: [2.82-4.85] **[63]**. An even more recent meta-analysis, including 10 studies, confirmed the association of this genetic anomaly with neonatal stroke **[53]**. Despite the large number of studies showing a high frequency of LVF in patients, studies showing a significant association with the disease remain limited **(tableVI) [27,55,28]**. Some studies have suggested a weak or non-existent link between LVF polymorphism and stroke in neonates **[5,38,51]**.
The involvement of this genetic anomaly in the pathogenesis of neonatal stroke remains controversial.

Table VI: Frequency of factor V Leiden polymorphism in neonatal ischemic stroke

Series		Factor V Leiden (%)	*p*	OR IC95%
Kurnik et al.	**[56]**	14,8		
Kenet et al.	**[63]**	15,3		3,75 [2,82-4,85]
Shatla et al.	**[55]**	25	-	-
Renaud et al.	**[64]**	3,5	>0,05	[0,7-9,9]
Duran et al.	**[78]**	23,3	<0.05	
Curtis et al.	**[51]**	6,3		6,3 [-0,7-17,9]
Simchen et al.	**[27]**	26,1		4,2 [1,5-11,3]

2-4-Mutation of the G20210A factor II gene

Prothrombin (Factor II) is the precursor of thrombin, a key enzyme in the coagulation cascade. Indeed, thrombin exerts procoagulant activities, converting fibrinogen to fibrin, activating factor XIII and amplifying its own formation. Mutation of the G20210A prothrombin gene is associated with high levels of factor II in plasma, and can only be detected by molecular biology. Studies carried out to date have not confirmed a correlation between the G20210A mutation and neonatal stroke **[64].**

The G20210A mutation in the factor II gene is a frequent hereditary prothrombotic anomaly that varies according to the ethnicity of populations. Its association with venous thromboembolic disease (VTE) has already been well established in the literature **[65]**. The absence of an association between this mutation and stroke in newborns has been noted in some recent studies **[38,50, 66]**. A meta-analysis of 13 studies revealed an OR of 2.60 IC95%: [1.66- 4.08] **[62]**. A more recent meta-analysis, including 10 studies, did not support a significant correlation between the G20210A mutation in the prothrombin gene and neonatal stroke **[53]**. In addition, the majority of studies reported frequencies of less than 10% (**Table VII**).

Table VII: Prothrombin gene mutation in neonatal ischemic stroke

Series		Factor II gene G20210A mutation (%)
Gefland et al	**[66]**	0
Shatla et al	**[55]**	5
Renaud	**[5]**	1,3
Curry et al	**[54]**	10
Curtis et al	**[51]**	2,2
Deveber et al	**[58]**	3,3

2-5-C677T polymorphism of the MTHFR gene

MTHFR is an important regulatory enzyme in the metabolism of folates (folic acid/vitamin B9 derivatives) and homocysteine **[67]**.
Several researchers have investigated the C677T polymorphism of the MTHFR gene and its involvement in neonatal stroke. Their results were heterogeneous **(Table VIII)** **[67, 68, 69]**. A Tunisian study by Oueslati **[52]** found the MTHFR mutation in 33.4% of cases. A recent study in North America revealed a fairly high prevalence of the MTHFR C677T polymorphism in stroke patients (CT and TT genotypes distributed 37.2% and 9.3% respectively), but this was not significantly different from that detected in controls (CT and TT genotypes distributed 37% and 15% respectively) **[51]**. The role of this polymorphism in the pathogenesis of deep vein thrombosis is well established. A direct consequence of MTHFR gene polymorphism is elevated blood homocysteine levels.
This hyperhomocysteinemia could be toxic to endothelial cells, leading to platelet activation and clot formation. In addition, a decrease in CP and AT

activity has been observed in hyperhomocysteinemia. The presence of high homocysteine levels in the blood could therefore create a favourable environment for venous thrombosis **[70, 71]**.

Table VIII: C677T polymorphism of the MTHFR gene in neonatal ischemic stroke

Series		MTHFR (%)			p or OR IC95%
			Heterozygous CT	Homozygous TT	
Gefland et al.	**[66]**	47	39	8	2.0 [0,6-6,8]
Shatla et al.	**[55]**	50	20	30	
Perez et al.	**[53]**		13,1		
Curry et al.	**[54]**	22	6	17	$p<0,05$
Simchen et al.	**[27]**	21,7		21,7	1,4 [0,6- 3,5]
Muwakkit et al.	**[50]**	54,2	41,7	12,5	$p>0.05$
Alsayouf et al.	**[67]**	8		8	$p>0,05$

2-6-Antiphospholipid antibodies

Three conventional types of antiphospholipid antibodies are defined: circulating anticoagulants (CCA) of the lupus anticoagulant (LA) type, anticardiolipins (aCL) and anti-beta-2-glycoprotein I (anti-β2GPI). These anti-phosphlipid antibodies are thought to be involved in venous thrombosis via two different mechanisms. Firstly, they interact with cellular phospholipids in platelets, leading to thrombocytopenia and subsequent activation of coagulation **[72]**.

On the other hand, these antibodies inhibit AT activity by binding to heparin sulfates.

A positive antiphospholipid test should be confirmed on a second sample taken 12 weeks apart **[73]**.

Antiphospholipid syndrome (APS) is defined by the presence of thrombosis (venous, arterial, microvascular, or a combination of these) and/or obstetric morbidity (miscarriage, preterm delivery, MFIU) with persistent anti-phospholipid antibody (aPL) positivity for at least 12 weeks. These aPL antibodies form a heterogeneous family, including LA-type ACCs, IgG or IgM-type anticardiolipin antibodies (aCL) and IgG or IgM-type anti-β2-glycoprotein I (anti-β2GPI) antibodies **[74]**. The aPLs recognize not only phospholipids but also serum proteins that are cofactors and can bind phospholipids (protein C, protein S, thrombomodulin, annexin and β2GPI) **[75]**. The pathophysiology of APAS is thus based on the disruption of the coagulation system towards a pro-coagulant state by interfering with coagulation regulators, activating cells involved in coagulation, inhibiting fibrinolysis and activating the complement system **[76]**.

The association of these antibodies with the onset of deep vein thrombosis and spontaneous abortion has already been confirmed in the literature. As a result, the newborns of mothers carrying SAPL would be more exposed to the risk of thromboembolic accidents and therefore perinatal stroke, given the passive transmission of these antibodies to the fetus during pregnancy. This hypothesis has been supported by some studies, which have found that newborns of mothers carrying SAPL have an increased risk of perinatal stroke. In our series, only one female newborn had a positive antiphospholipid antibody test. The same result was reported by Munoz et al **[38]**. Furthermore, in a recent Canadian study, all patients tested negative for antiphospholipid antibodies **[51]**.

However, the results of studies into the role of these antibodies in triggering perinatal stroke remain controversial. Indeed, some studies have shown that antiphospholipid antibodies are significantly linked to the disease **[27]**. For example, a meta-analysis of 8 studies showed a strong association between antiphospholipid antibodies and stroke, with an OR=6.95 and CI95% [3.67-13.14] **[77]**. On the other hand, other studies, despite a high positivity rate for these antibodies, were unable to establish this association. Such is the case of the study by Duran et al. in which they reported a prevalence of type LA antiphospholipids of the order of 16.7% in neonatal stroke, but without a statistically significant association **[78]**. Another study, including 62 neonates with strokei, revealed positive type LA ACC in 12 neonates. However, after regular monitoring, these levels normalized in 10 children within an average of two and a half years. The authors concluded that antiphospholipids were not a risk factor for stroke **[79]**.

2-7- Place of combined coagulation anomalies

In an Egyptian study by Shatla et al, coagulation anomalies were combined in 20% of cases. **[55]**.

Kurnik et al. also found a percentage of 14.4% of combined pro-thrombotic anomalies. More than that, their study showed that the risk of recurrent stroke is increased in children with associated coagulation abnormalities **[56]**.

According to the literature, the combination of prothrombotic anomalies affects between 11.1% and 30% of newborns with stroke.

2-8- Role of lipoprotein 'a' in the onset of ischemic stroke in neonates

According to recent studies, the risk of neonatal stroke is increased for the presence of Vleiden factor polymorphism, MTHFR polymorphism and elevated Lp 'a' **[70, 80]**.

In fact, Lp 'a' competes with plasminogen due to their close structural relationship, thus linking this lipoprotein to the proteins of the haemostasis system. This anomaly is considered a genetic risk factor in young adults, confirmed by a recent meta-analysis. In addition, high Lp 'a' concentrations have been found in neonates with iCVA and in their mothers, acting synergistically with other prothrombotic abnormalities **[53]**.

The latter represents an acquired comorbidity factor, increasing the risk of stroke, particularly when other thrombophilic risk factors coexist. For this reason, Lp 'a' assays should be requested, in addition to the search for FVL and MTHFR mutations in etiological work-ups.

EXAMINATIONS ADDITIONAL

VI- FURTHER TESTS

Imaging plays a central role in the diagnosis of neonatal cerebral infarction, to authenticate arterial ischemia, specify its topography and extent and, in some cases, assess the time of onset. When faced with an acute neonatal neurological picture, it can help rule out other pathological causes and guide the implementation of specific therapies. It also provides prognostic information both during the acute period and when assessing lesions at a distance from the episode **[81,82]**.

Three exploration techniques are used.

1- Transfontanellar ultrasound and Doppler

It's an available, harmless test. It can be performed at the patient's bedside, even in unstable newborns or those on ventilatory support. It can be repeated without restriction, and remains the primary method for examining the neonatal brain prior to any complementary secondary exploration. However, there are a number of limitations. Typical ischemic events are clearly visible. They take the form of triangular hyperechogenicity with a cortical base, typically well limited and involving the cortex and subcortical white matter, with loss of definition of adjacent convolutions corresponding to an arterial territory **[83,57]**.

2- Cerebral computed tomography

It is a rapid exploration tool that highlights the stroke, its location and extent, although it is not ideal for exploring the posterior fossa. Cerebral computed tomography (CT) accurately reveals superficial or hemorrhagic lesions not detected by ETF.

CT is generally performed at the acute stage without injection of contrast medium **[83,57]**.

3- Magnetic resonance imaging

Like ETF, MRI does not expose the newborn to the potentially harmful effects of ionizing radiation. MRI is the examination of choice for assessing brain parenchyma in term newborns. In the case of stroke, it is the most sensitive and early technique. It enables analysis of lesion topography: arterial or non-arterial distribution, involvement of junctional zones. The basic protocol for newborns includes T1-, T2-, diffusion-, angio-MRI- and T1-weighted sequences after intravenous injection of gadolinium **[84]**.

VII- GENERAL ASSESSMENT OF ISCHEMIC STROKE IN NEWBORNS

Once the diagnosis of stroke in a newborn has been confirmed, an etiological work-up is recommended to determine the risk factors involved in the disease.

This etiological assessment aims to :

- Investigate maternal, obstetric and neonatal risk factors.
- Search for an arterial vascular anomaly (thrombosis / dissection / congenital hypoplasia...) by cervico-cerebral angio-MRI if not already performed or, failing that, Doppler ultrasound of the supra-aortic trunks.
- Search for congenital emboligenic heart disease with a echocardiography.
- Investigate coagulation abnormalities by means of biological coagulation tests.

We propose an approach to the etiological investigation of stroke in newborns (**figure 4**).

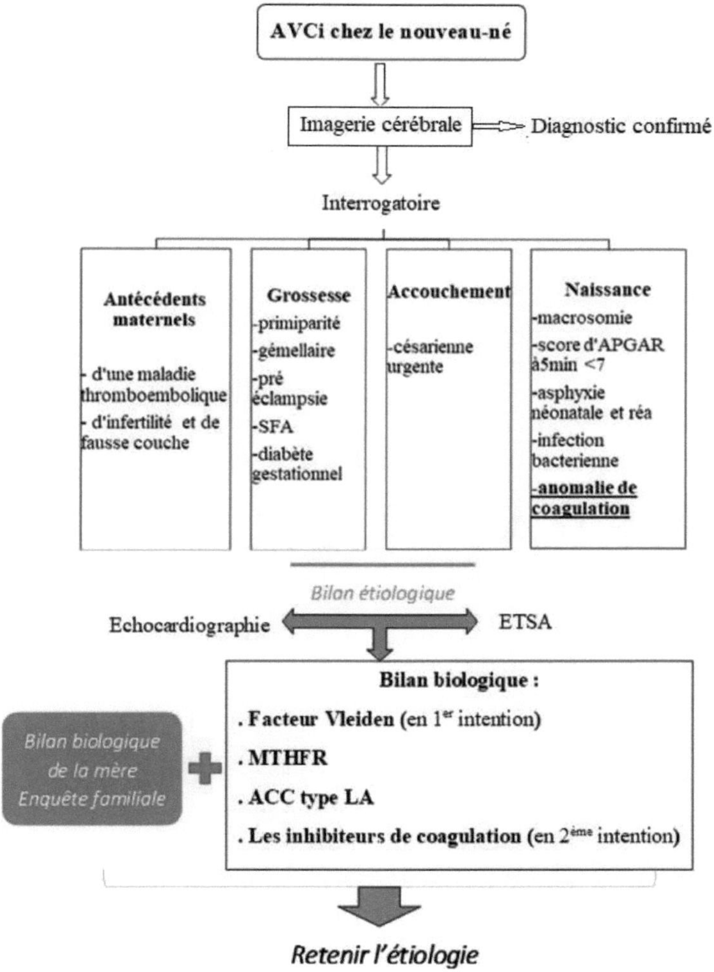

AVCi chez le nouveau-né

Imagerie cérébrale → Diagnostic confirmé

Interrogatoire

Antécédents maternels
- d'une maladie thromboembolique
- d'infertilité et de fausse couche

Grossesse
-primiparité
-gémellaire
-pré éclampsie
-SFA
-diabète gestationnel

Accouchement
-césarienne urgente

Naissance
-macrosomie
-score d'APGAR à5min <7
-asphyxie néonatale et réa
-infection bacterienne
-anomalie de coagulation

Bilan étiologique

Echocardiographie ↔ ETSA

Bilan biologique :
. **Facteur Vleiden** (en 1er intention)
. **MTHFR**
. **ACC type LA**
. **Les inhibiteurs de coagulation** (en 2ème intention)

Bilan biologique de la mère
Enquête familiale

Retenir l'étiologie

Figure 4: Assessment of ischemic stroke in newborns

CARE THERAPEUTICS

VIII- CARE

1- Therapeutic management in the acute phase

The recurrence rate of arterial stroke in neonates, other than those with congenital heart disease or thrombophilia, is very low (<1%), in contrast to stroke in older children or adults. Thus, the use of thrombolytics or anticoagulants, including heparin or antiplatelet agents, is not recommended in neonates **[85]**.

During the acute phase, the main symptomatic treatment is for seizures. Indeed, seizures resulting from stroke generally respond well to standard anticonvulsant medication. Although still widely debated, intervention is required in cases of status epilepticus, clinical seizures lasting more than 5 consecutive minutes, or shorter (> 30 seconds) but repeated seizures (2 or more per hour) **[23]**.

Phenobarbital remains the most frequently prescribed drug for the initial treatment of neonatal convulsions. Indeed, it is the drug with which clinicians have the most experience. Its dosage is as follows: loading dose of 20 mg/kg given by intravenous infusion over 20 minutes, followed, if necessary, by a second loading dose (10 mg/kg) to achieve a barbitemia of 25-30 mg/L. It is advisable to use a single antiepileptic drug at its maximum dosage, and in the event of recurrence, to propose a combination with an antiepileptic drug with a different mechanism of action **[86]**.

Phenobarbital should be used as first-line treatment, followed by phenytoin if this fails, then clonazepam **[24]**. Other objectives are to correct acid-base imbalance and electrolyte abnormalities, ensure adequate oxygenation and ventilation, treat anemia and provide antibiotic therapy in the event of bacterial infection **[4]**. The *American College of Chest Physicians* (ACCP) suggests that only neonates with first-episode arterial stroke and a proven cardioembolic etiology should receive treatment with unfractionated heparin or low-molecular-weight heparin, but any anticoagulant or aspirin therapy has been discouraged in neonates with non-cardioembolic arterial stroke **[87]**.

2- Functional support

Progression in the first few months is usually straightforward. Seizures are generally easily controlled by initial treatment. Following a neonatal stroke, the child's development may be complicated by various motor and cognitive sequelae. Motor deficits may manifest themselves in children during the first few months as cerebral palsy **[88]**.

As soon as the acute phase of stroke has been resolved, interventional rehabilitation therapy should be started **[89]**. The aim of early rehabilitation with physiotherapy, occupational therapy or psychomotor therapy (separately or in combination) is to maintain joint amplitudes and avoid orthopedic deformities **[90]**.

Then, these measures must be combined with a more global intervention with the child, enabling him to carry out his activities and, above all, to integrate socially despite his deficit syndrome. After-effects must be detected and monitored. A multidisciplinary approach involving pediatricians, physical physicians, physiotherapists, occupational therapists, speech therapists, speech therapists, neuropediatricians, child psychiatrists and ophthalmologists is required to optimize functional performance, promote rehabilitation and generally improve quality of life.

CONCLUSION

Perinatal ischemic stroke is the most frequent form of pediatric stroke. It is due to a focal interruption of cerebral blood flow, occurring between 20ème gestational weeks.

and the 28ème day of life. Its incidence varies from one study to another, depending on inclusion and exclusion criteria.

Perinatal ischemic stroke is a multifactorial event resulting from the interaction of several acquired or constitutional determinants, concerning the mother, the fetus and the placenta. The presence of thrombophilia disorders In fact, the hemostasis of the newborn embodies a developing system, with its players showing functional and quantitative modifications during the first months of life, which must be mastered by clinicians and biologists in order to direct a correct etiological diagnosis and adequate patient management.

Given the complexity of the pathophysiology of neonatal stroke, a comprehensive and targeted etiological investigation is of great value in improving the quality of life of these children and their parents.

Following a neonatal stroke, the child's development may be complicated by various motor and cognitive sequelae. Motor deficits may manifest themselves in children during the first few months as cerebral palsy. The aim of early rehabilitation using physiotherapy, occupational therapy or psychomotricity (separately or in combination) is to maintain joint amplitudes and avoid orthopedic deformities.

Secondly, these measures must be combined with a more global intervention with techild, enabling him to carry out his activities and, above all, to integrate socially despite his deficit syndrome.

REFERENCES

1. **Azcona B, Layouni I.** Perinatal cerebrovascular accidents. *Med Ther Pediatr.2011;14:238-45.*

2. **Ngoma Souamy ML.** Les Textilomes intrapéritonéaux à propos de 2 cas avec revue de la littérature [Thesis]. *Rabat: Université Mohammed V-Souissi, Faculté de Médecine et de Pharmacie;. 2013.*

3. **Adami RR, Grundy ME, Poretti A, Felling RJ, Lemmon M, Graham EM.** Distinguishing arterial ischemic stroke from hypoxic-ischemic encephalo-pathy in the neonate at birth. *Obstet Gynecol.2016;128:704-12.*

4. **Ferriero DM, Fullerton HJ, Bernard TJ, Billinghurst L, Daniels SR, DeBaun MR, et al.** Management of stroke in neonates and children: a scientific statement from the American Heart Association/American Stroke Association. *Stroke.2019;50:e51-e96.*

5. **Renaud C.** Cerebral arterial infarction in term newborns: clinical presentation, risk factors and evolutionary determinants from a prospective multicenter descriptive epidemiology cohort [Thesis]. *Saint Etienne: Université Jean Monnet; 2011.*

6. **National Reference Center for Childhood Stroke.** Les Maladies. *[Online]. 2019 [Accessed 24/12/2022], available at URL: http://www.cnravcenfant.fr/AVC_Phase_Aigue/Maladies/Les_Maladies.htm l*

7. **deVeber GA, Kirton A, Booth FA, Yager JY, Wirrell EC, Wood E, et al.** Epidemiology and outcomes of arterial ischemic stroke in children: The Canadian Pediatric Ischemic Stroke Registry. *Pediatr Neurol.2017;69:58-70.*

8. **Darmency-Stamboul V, Cordier AG, Chabrier S.** Arterial ischemic stroke in term and near-term neonates: prevalence and risk factors. *Arch Pediatr.2017;24:9S3-11.*

9. **Dunbar M, Kirton A.** Perinatal Stroke. *Semin Pediatr Neurol. 2019;32: 100767.*

10. **Dunbar M, Mineyko A, Hill M, Hodge J, Floer A, Kirton A.**

Population based birth prevalence of disease-specific perinatal stroke. *Pediatrics. 2020;146:e2020013201.*

11. **Golomb MR, Fullerton HJ, Nowak-Gottl U, Deveber G.** Male predominance in childhood ischemic stroke: findings from the international pediatric stroke study. *Stroke. 2009;40:52-7.*

12. **Wagenaar N, Martinez-Biarge M, van der Aa NE, van Haastert IC, Groenendaal F, Benders MJ, et al.** Neurodevelopment after perinatal arterial ischemic stroke. *Pediatrics.2018;142:e20174164.*

13. Rhee CJ, da Costa CS, Austin T, Brady KM, Czosnyka M, Lee JK. Neonatal cerebrovascular autoregulation. *Pediatr Res. 2018;84:602-10.*

14. **Chabrier S, Husson B, Dinomais M, Landrieu P, Nguyen The Tich S.** New insights (and new interrogations) in perinatal arterial ischemic stroke. *Thromb Res. 2011;127:13-22.*

15. **Stago.** History of Thrombosis. *[Online]. [Accessed 29/08/2022], available at URL: https://www.stago.com/fr/lhemostase/histoire-de-la-thrombose/*

16. **Robert J.** Evaluation of the PERC score and YEARS algorithm in the diagnosis of pulmonary embolism: a retrospective study in the emergency department of Caen University Hospital [Thesis]. *Cean: Université de Caen - Normandie, Faculté de Médecine; 2018.*

17. **Martinez-Biarge M, Ferriero DM, Cowan FM.** Perinatal arterial ischemic stroke. *Handb Clin Neurol. 2019;162:239-66.*

18. **Nouri-Merchaoui S, Mahdhaoui N, Trabelsi S, Seboui H.** Neonatal arterial thrombosis not caused by arterial catheterization: about 4 observations. *Arch Pediatr. 2012;19:413-8.*

19. **Roy B, Arbuckle S, Walker K, Morgan C, Galea C, Badawi N, et al.** The role of the placenta in perinatal stroke: a systematic review. *J Child Neurol. 2020;35:773-83.*

20. Finnemore A, Groves A. Physiology of the fetal and transitional circulation.

Semin Fetal Neonatal Med. 2015;20:210-6.

21. **Kara-Zaitri MA.** Fetal circulation. *[Online]. 2021 [Accessed 07/11/2022], Available from URL: https://www.dr-karazaitri-ma.net/embryology/fetal-circulation-2/*

22. **Hamida N, Hakim A, Fourati H, Ben Thabet A, Walha L, Bouraoui A, et al.** Neonatal cervical arterial dissection secondary to obstetrical trauma. *Arch Pediatr. 2014;21:201-5.*

23. **Saliba E, Debillon T, Auvin S, Baud O, Biran V, Chabernaud JL, et al.** Neonatal arterial ischemic stroke: summary of recommendations. *Arch Pediatr. 2017;24:180-8.*

24. **Klučka J, Klabusayová E, Musilová T, Kramplová T, Skříšovská T, Kratochvíl M, et al.** Pediatric patient with ischemic stroke: initial approach and early management. *Children (Basel). 2021;8:649.*

25. **Amlie-Lefond C.** Evaluation and acute management of ischemic stroke in infants and children. *Continuum (Minneap Minn). 2018;24:150-70.*

26. **Chabrier S, Kossorotoff M, Chevin M, Fluss J.** Perinatal stroke: nosography, clinical presentation, pathogenesis, risk factors and genetics. *Bull Acad Nat Med. 2021;205:490-8.*

27. **Simchen MJ, Goldstein G, Lubetsky A, Strauss T, Schiff E, Kenet G.** Factor v Leiden and antiphospholipid antibodies in either mothers or infants increase the risk for perinatal arterial ischemic stroke. *Stroke. 2009;40:65-70.*

28. **Arnaez J, Arca G, Martín-Ancel A, Agut T, Garcia-Alix A.** Neonatal arterial ischemic stroke: risk related to family history, maternal diseases, and genetic thrombophilia. *Clin Appl Thromb. 2018;24:79-84.*

29. **Kopyta I, Cebula A, Sarecka-Hujar B.** Early deaths after arterial ischemic stroke in pediatric patients: incidence and risk factors. *Children*

(Basel). 2021;8:471.

30. **Poon LC, Shennan A, Hyett JA, Kapur A, Hadar E, Divakar H, et al.** The International Federation of Gynecology and Obstetrics (FIGO) initiative on pre-eclampsia: A pragmatic guide for first-trimester screening and prevention. *Int J Gynecol Obstet. 2019;145:1-33.*

31. **Felling RJ, Sun LR, Maxwell EC, Goldenberg N, Bernard T.** Pediatric arterial ischemic stroke: Epidemiology, risk factors, and management. *Blood Cells Mol Dis. 2017;67:23-33..*

32. **Dueck CC, Grynspan D, Eisenstat DD, Caces R, Rafay MF.** Ischemic perinatal stroke secondary to chorioamnionitis: a histopathological case presentation. *J Child Neurol. 2009;24:1557-60.*

33. **Chabrier S, Saliba E, Nguyen The Tich S, Charollais A, Varlet MN, Tardy B, et al.** Obstetrical and neonatal characteristics vary with birthweight in a cohort of 100 term newborns with symptomatic arterial ischemic stroke. *Eur J Paediatr Neurol. 2010;14:206-13.*

34. **Sorg AL, von Kries R, Klemme M, Gerstl L, Weinberger R, Beyerlein A, et al.** Risk factors for perinatal arterial ischaemic stroke: a large case-control study. *Dev Med Child Neurol. 2020;62:513-20*

35. **Sutherly LJ, Malloy R.** Risk factors of pediatric stroke. *J Neurosci Nurs. 2020;52:58-60.*

36. **Kamate M, Reddy NA, Detroja M.** Perinatal infections: an important etiological risk factor for mineralizing angiopathy. *Indian J Pediatr. 2021; 88:58-60*

37. **Li C, Miao JK, Xu Y, Hua YY, Ma Q, Zhou LL, et al.** Prenatal, perinatal and neonatal risk factors for perinatal arterial ischaemic stroke: a systematic review and meta-analysis. *Eur J Neurol. 2017;24:1006-15.*

38. **Munoz D, Hidalgo MJ, Balut F, Troncoso M, Lara S, Barrios A, et al.** Risk factors for perinatal arterial ischemic stroke: a case-control study. *Cell*

Med. 2018;10:1-6.

39. **Darmency-Stamboul V, Chantegret C, Ferdynus C, Mejean N, Durand C, Sagot P, et al.** Antenatal factors associated with perinatal arterial ischemic stroke. *Stroke. 2012;43:2307-12*

40. **Giraud A, Guiraut C, Chevin M, Chabrier S, Sébire G.** Role of perinatal inflammation in neonatal arterial ischemic stroke. *Front Neurol. 2017;8: 612.*

41. **Kharoubi S, Bastandji A, Ahmouda W, Bounour D, Bouslama F, Layachi F, et al.** SFP-P106 - Emergencies - Laryngeal respiratory emergencies in the pediatric setting in Algeria. *Arch Pediatr. 2008;15:975.*

42. **Harteman JC, Groenendaal F, Kwee A, Welsing PM, Benders MJ, de Vries LS.** Risk factors for perinatal arterial ischaemic stroke in full-term infants: a case-control study. *Arch Dis Child Fetal Neonatal Ed. 2012;97:F411-6.*

43. **Barnes C, Deveber G.** Prothrombotic abnormalities in childhood ischaemic stroke. *Thromb Res. 2006;118:67-74.*

44. **Lejus C, Pajot S, Le Roux C, Surbled M.** Hemostasis in the newborn: what the clinician needs to know. *Arch Pediatr. 2010;17:862-3.*

45. **Periayah MH, Halim AS, Mat Saad AZ.** Mechanism action of platelets and crucial blood coagulation pathways in hemostasis. *Int J Hematol Oncol Stem Cell Res. 2017;11:319-27.*

46. **de Revel T.** Physiology of hemostasis. *EMC-Dentistry. 2004;1:71-81.*

47. **Rey E, Kahn SR, David M, Shrier I.** Thrombophilic disorders and fetal loss: a meta-analysis. *Lancet. 2003;361:901-8.*

48. **Nelson KB.** Thrombophilias, perinatal stroke, and cerebral palsy. *Clin Obstet Gynecol. 2006;49:875-84.*

49. **Arboix A, Jiménez C, Massons J, Parra O, Besses C.** Hematological disorders: a commonly unrecognized cause of acute stroke. *Expert Rev*

Hematol. 2016;9:891-901.

***50.* Muwakkit SA, Majdalani M, Hourani R, Mahfouz RA, Otrock ZK, Bilalian C, et al.** Inherited thrombophilia in childhood arterial stroke: data from Lebanon. *Pediatr Neurol. 2011;45:155-8.*

***51.* Curtis C, Mineyko A, Massicotte P, Leaker M, Jiang XY, Floer A, et al.** Thrombophilia risk is not increased in children after perinatal stroke. *Blood. 2017;129:2793-800.*

***52.* Oueslati I.** Arterial and venous thromboembolic vascular accidents of the ante- and postnatal periods: about 11 cases [Thesis]. *Monastir: University of Monastir, Faculty of Pharmacy; 2013.*

***53.* Perez T, Valentin Jb, Saliba E, Gruel Y.** Ischemic stroke in the newborn: which biological thrombotic risk factors to look for and what are the consequences in practice? *Arch Pediatr. 2017;24:9S28-34.*

***54.* Curry CJ, Bhullar S, Holmes J, Delozier CD, Roeder ER, Hutchison HT.** Risk factors for perinatal arterial stroke: a study of 60 mother-child pairs. *Pediatr Neurol. 2007;37:99-107.*

***55.* Shatla HM, Tomoum HY, Elsayed SM, Aly RH, Shatla RH, Ismail MA, et al.** Inherited thrombophilia in pediatric ischemic stroke: an Egyptian study. *Pediatr Neurol. 2012;47:114-8.*

***56.* Kurnik K, Kosch A, Sträter R, Schobess R, Heller C, Nowak-Göttl U.** Recurrent thromboembolism in infants and children suffering from symptomatic neonatal arterial stroke: a prospective follow-up study. *Stroke. 2003;34:2887-92.*

***57.* Husson B, Durand C, Hertz-Pannier L.** Recommendations for imaging ischemic stroke in the newborn. *Arch Pediatr. 2017;24:9S19-27.*

***58.* deVeber G, Kirkham F, Shannon K, Brandão L, Sträter R, Kenet G, et al.** Recurrent stroke: the role of thrombophilia in a large international pediatric stroke population. *Haematologica. 2019;104:1676-81.*

***59.* Sirachainan N, Limrungsikul A, Chuansumrit A, Nuntnarumit P, Thampratankul L, Wangruangsathit S, et al.** Incidences, risk factors and outcomes of neonatal thromboembolism. *J Matern Fetal Neonatal Med. 2018;31:347-51.*

***60.* Colvin BT.** Physiology of haemostasis. *Vox Sang. 2004;87:43-6.*

***61.* Charvier A.** Prescription of thrombophilia workup in the presence of venous thromboembolic disease and therapeutic consequences: evaluation of practices in general practice (Languedoc- Roussillon region) [Thesis]. *Montpellier: University of Montpellier, Faculty of Medicine; 2018.*

***62.* M'barek L, Sakka S, Meghdiche F, Turki D, Maalla K, Dammak M, et al.** MTHFR (C677T, A1298C), FV Leiden polymorphisms, and the prothrombin G20210A mutation in arterial ischemic stroke among young Tunisian adults. *Metab Brain Dis. 2021;36:421- 8.*

***63.* Kenet G, Lütkhoff LK, Albisetti M, Bernard T, Bonduel M, Brandao L, et al.** Impact of thrombophilia on risk of arterial ischemic stroke or cerebral sinovenous thrombosis in neonates and children: a systematic review and meta-analysis of observational studies. *Circulation. 2010;121:1838-47.*

***64.* Renaud C, Tardy-Poncet B, Presles E, Chabrier S.** Low prevalence of coagulation F2 and F5 polymorphisms in mothers and children in a large cohort of patients with neonatal arterial ischemic stroke. *Br J Haematol. 2010;150:709-12.*

***65.* Mokhtar Ahmed A, Rishaorcid AI, El-Taher AK, Abdelhy RM, AbdElmonem DM.** Impact of factor v Leiden G1691A, MTHFR C677T, and prothrombin G20210 a mutations on the development of neonatal thrombosis. *Zagazig Univ Med J. 2022;28:1156-63.*

***66.* Gelfand AA, Croen LA, Torres AR, Wu YW.** Genetic risk factors for perinatal arterial ischemic stroke. *Pediatr Neurol. 2013;48:36-41.*

***67.* Alsayouf H, Zamel KM, Heyer GL, Khuhro AL, Kahwash SB, de los**

Reyes EC. Role of methylenetetrahydrofolate reductase gene (MTHFR) 677C>T polymorphism in pediatric cerebrovascular disorders. *J Child Neurol. 2011;26:318-21.*

68. **Leclerc D, Rozen R.** Molecular genetics of MTHFR: not all polymorphisms are benign. *Med Sci (Paris). 2007;23:297-302.*

69. **Hickey SE, Curry CJ, Toriello HV.** ACMG practice guideline: lack of evidence for MTHFR polymorphism testing. *Genet Med. 2013;15:153-6.*

70. **Coen Herak D, Lenicek Krleza J, Radic Antolic M, Horvat I, Djuranovic V, Zrinski Topic R, et al.** Association of polymorphisms in coagulation factor genes and enzymes of homocysteine metabolism with arterial ischemic stroke in children. *Clin Appl Thromb Hemost. 2017;23:1042-51.*

71. **Khalil AM, Al Banna EA, Huwas ZS, Abd Almonem DM.** Role of thrombophilia in neonatal thrombosis as a risk factor. *Egypt J Hosp Med. 2021;84:2605-11*

72. **Mekinian A, Lachassinne E, Nicaise-Roland P, Carbillon L, Motta M, Vicaut E, et al.** European registry of babies born to mothers with antiphospholipid syndrome. *Ann Rheum Dis. 2013;72:217-22.*

73. **Ramaharo-Ratiarison D.** Clinico-biological profiles associated with the presence of low-intensity anticoagulant lupus: which management to adopt? [Thesis]. *Bordeaux: Université de Bordeaux, U.F.R des Sciences Médicales; 2018.*

74. **Cohen H, Efthymiou M, Gates C, Isenberg D.** Direct oral anticoagulants for thromboprophylaxis in patients with antiphospholipid syndrome. *Semin Thromb Hemost. 2018;44:427-38.*

75. **Radin M, Cecchi I, Foddai SG, Rubini E, Barinotti A, Ramirez C, et al.** Validation of the particle-based multi-analyte technology for detection of Anti-PhosphatidylSerine/Prothrombin antibodies. *Biomedicines. 2020; 8:622.*

76. **Sciascia S, Amigo MC, Roccatello D, Khamashta M.** Diagnosing antiphospholipid syndrome: "extra-criteria" manifestations and technical advances. *Nat Rev Rheumatol. 2017;13:548-60*

77. **Sarecka-Hujar B, Kopyta I.** Risk factors for recurrent arterial ischemic stroke in children and young adults. *Brain Sci. 2020;10:24.*

78. **Duran R, Biner B, Demir M, Çeltik C, Karasalihoğlu S.** Factor v Leiden mutation and other thrombophilia markers in childhood ischemic stroke. *Clin Appl Thromb. 2005;11:83-8.*

79. **Berkun Y, Simchen M, Strauss T, Menashcu S, Padeh S, Kenet G.** Antiphospholipid antibodies in neonates with stroke - a unique entity or variant of antiphospholipid syndrome? *Lupus. 2014;23:986-93.*

80. **Nowak-Göttl U, Langer C, Bergs S, Thedieck S, Sträter R, Stoll M.** Genetics of hemostasis: differential effects of heritability and household components influencing lipid concentrations and clotting factor levels in 282 pediatric stroke families. *Environ Health Perspect. 2008;116:839-43.*

81. **Nguyen The Tich S.** Place of electroencephalogram in the management of arterial ischemic stroke in the newborn. *Arch Pediatr. 2017;24:9S41-5.*

82. **Srivastava R, Rajapakse T, Carlson HL, Keess J, Wei XC, Kirton A.** Diffusion imaging of cerebral diaschisis in neonatal arterial ischemic stroke. *Pediatr Neurol. 2019;100:49-54.*

83. **Maller VV, Choudhri AF, Cohen HL.** Neonatal head ultrasound: a review and update-part 2: the term neonate and analysis of brain anomalies. *Ultrasound Q. 2019;35:212-23.*

84. **Biswas A, Mankad K, Shroff M, Hanagandi P, Krishnan P.** Neuroimaging perspectives of perinatal arterial ischemic stroke. *Pediatr Neurol. 2020;113:56-65.*

85. **Debillon T, de Launay C, Ego A.** Recommendations for the management of neonatal-onset cerebral arterial infarction in term or near-term neonates. *Arch Pediatr. 2017;24:9S1-2.*

***86.* Baud O, Auvin S, Saliba E, Biran V.** Therapeutic management of seizures associated with newborn stroke and prospects for neuroprotection in the acute phase. *Arch Pediatr. 2017;24: 9S46-50.*

***87.* Whitaker EE, Cipolla MJ.** Perinatal stroke. *Handb Clin Neurol. 2020; 171:313-26.*

***88.* Dinomais M, Marret S, Vuillerot C.** Cerebral plasticity and early rehabilitative management of children after neonatal arterial cerebral infarction. *Arch Pediatr. 2017;24:9S61-8.*

***89.* López-Espejo MA, Chávez MH, Huete I.** Short-term outcomes after a neonatal arterial ischemic stroke. *Childs Nerv Syst. 2021;37:1249-54.*

***90.* Makatsariya A, Bitsadze V, Khizroeva J, Vorobev A, Makatsariya N, Egorova E, et al.** Neonatal thrombosis. *J Matern Fetal Neonatal Med. 2022;35:1169-77.*

***91.* Machado V, Pimentel S, Pinto F, Nona J.** Perinatal ischemic stroke: a five- year retrospective study in a level-III maternity hospital. *Einstein (Sao Paulo). 2015;13:65-71.*

***92.* Grunt S, Mazenauer L, Buerki SE, Boltshauser E, Mori AC, Datta AN, et al.** Incidence and outcomes of symptomatic neonatal arterial ischemic stroke. *Pediatrics. 2015;135:e1220-8.*

***93.* Salih MA, Abdel-Gader AG, Al-Jarallah AA, Kentab AY, Alorainy IA, Hassan HH, et al.** Stroke in Saudi children. Epidemiology, clinical features and risk factors. *Saudi Med J. 2006;27:S12-20.*

***94.* Martinez-Biarge M, Cheong JL, Diez-Sebastian J, Mercuri E, Dubowitz LM, Cowan FM.** Risk factors for neonatal arterial ischemic stroke: the importance of the intrapartum period. *J Pediatr. 2016;173:62-8.*

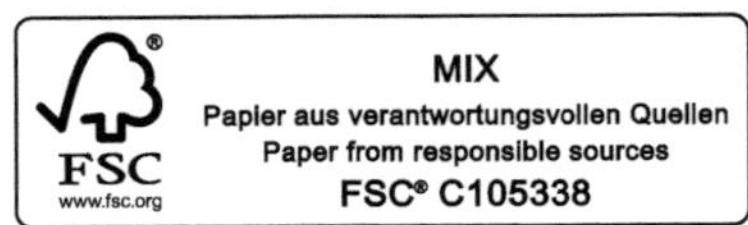

Printed by Books on Demand GmbH, Norderstedt / Germany